Amjed BEN HAOUALA
Najla SGHAIER

A neurobiological approach to gambling

Amjed BEN HAOUALA
Najla SGHAIER

A neurobiological approach to gambling

through a literature review

ScienciaScripts

Imprint

Any brand names and product names mentioned in this book are subject to trademark, brand or patent protection and are trademarks or registered trademarks of their respective holders. The use of brand names, product names, common names, trade names, product descriptions etc. even without a particular marking in this work is in no way to be construed to mean that such names may be regarded as unrestricted in respect of trademark and brand protection legislation and could thus be used by anyone.

Cover image: www.ingimage.com

This book is a translation from the original published under ISBN 978-620-6-73032-3.

Publisher:
Sciencia Scripts
is a trademark of
Dodo Books Indian Ocean Ltd. and OmniScriptum S.R.L publishing group

120 High Road, East Finchley, London, N2 9ED, United Kingdom
Str. Armeneasca 28/1, office 1, Chisinau MD-2012, Republic of Moldova, Europe
Managing Directors: Ieva Konstantinova, Victoria Ursu
info@omniscriptum.com

Printed at: see last page
ISBN: 978-620-8-64153-5

Copyright © Amjed BEN HAOUALA, Najla SGHAIER
Copyright © 2025 Dodo Books Indian Ocean Ltd. and OmniScriptum S.R.L publishing group

TABLE OF CONTENTS

INTRODUCTION

Gambling involves betting something of value (usually money) on an event whose outcome is uncertain, in the hope of winning a greater reward (1). Games are ubiquitous in many cultures and are becoming an increasingly important part of leisure activities (2). Popular forms of gambling include casino games (including table games, such as blackjack, and electronic games, such as slot machines), lotteries (including instant lotteries or scratch cards) and internet games (including poker or sports games) (3).

Although gambling is a recreational activity for most people, some gamblers lose control and gamble excessively, with dramatic financial, personal and professional consequences. Gambling Disorder is currently recognised as a psychiatric disorder in the fifth version of the Diagnostic and Statistical Manual of Mental Disorders (DSM-5) (4).

These numerous clinical, neurobiological and neuropsychological similarities with substance addiction have led the psychiatric community to redefine pathological gambling as a behavioural addiction, meeting precise criteria (4). Its prevalence is between 1 and 2% in Western countries. (5). These estimates are several times higher in adolescents and young adults (6).

Recent studies on pathological gambling suggest that prevalence estimates may increase due to greater availability of gambling in relation to changes in legislation, greater social acceptability and the recent liberalisation of certain online games (7).Over the last decade, considerable progress has been made in understanding the neurobiological basis of this disorder, particularly with the advent of neuroimaging. Several neurotransmitter systems (norepinephrine, serotonin, dopamine, opioids and glutamate) and brain regions (ventral striatum, ventromedial prefrontal cortex, insula, among others) have been implicated in pathological gambling (8).

A better understanding of the neurobiological mechanisms of this behavioural addiction therefore seems important for developing more targeted prevention and treatment strategies.Hence the interest of our study, the aim of which is illustrate through a review of the literature on the neurobiological basis of pathological gambling.

METHODOLOGY

I. Type of study

A systematic review of the literature was carried out using the Prisma-P methodology (the Preferred Reporting Items for Systematic Review and Meta-Analysis). Bibliographic reference sources were managed using Zotero software.

II. Procedure

1. Identification : exporting references to Zotero

The search equations were entered into Pubmed using the following terms: "Neurobiology", "Gambling Disorder", "Pathological Gambling", "Gambling" with the following formula: [Neurobiology] AND ["Gambling Disorder" OR "Pathological Gambling" OR "Gambling"].

The research was carried out from 1997 to 2024 identified 208 references.

2. Selection stage: Identification and removal of duplicates

After excluding duplicates, 202 references were retained.

3. Selection stage : selection and verification of articles on the basis of title and abstract

This stage consists of selecting articles on the basis of inclusion and exclusion criteria. The inclusion criteria are clinical trials, randomised controlled trials and systematic reviews published between 1997 and 2024, the primary or secondary objectives of which were study the various neurobiological mechanisms of pathological gambling. We did not use a restriction in relation to the publication date.

4. Eligibility : Assessment of item's eligibility in full text

At this stage, the analysis of the eligibility of articles is based on the evaluation of the inclusion and exclusion criteria by reading the entire text. The eligibility process was similar to that used for the initial selection, based on the title and abstract. In the end, only 27 articles met our criteria and were included in our study. To summarise these four stages, a PRISMA flow diagram has been drawn up.

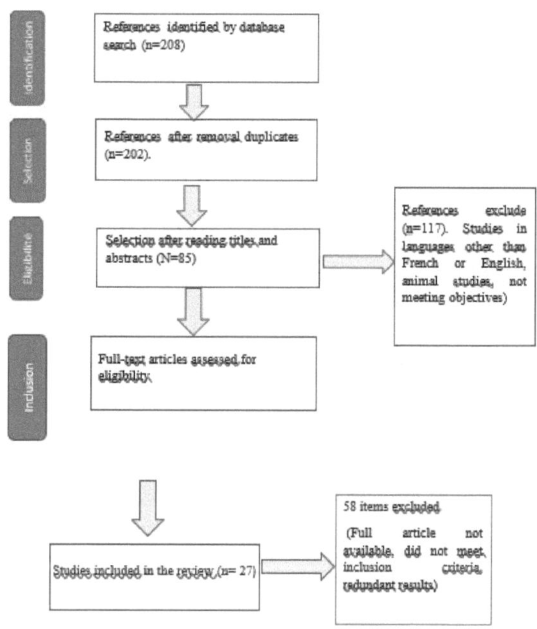

RESULTS

Our work included 27 articles dealing with the neurobiology of pathological gambling. These articles explore mechanisms from a neuroimaging and neurochemical perspective. Other articles explore the therapeutic implications of these mechanisms in pathological gambling.

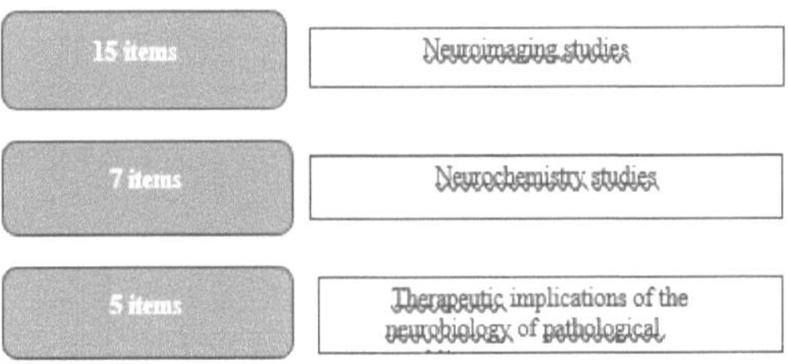

I. The gambling pathological at as addiction in the DSM-5 :

Pathological gambling has long been considered an "impulse control disorder" in DSM-3 and DSM-4 (9). It is now redefined as an addiction in the DSM-5 (Figure 1), making it the first and only behavioural addiction (non-substance-related disorder) to be officially recognised (4). In the DSM-5, pathological gambling (also known as gambling disorder) is defined by a pattern of "maladaptive, persistent and repeated gambling behaviour" that disrupts various personal, family and professional domains. To make the diagnosis, at least four of nine criteria must be present over a twelve-month period (Figure 1). Gambling problem which occurs mainly during a manic episode is an exclusion criterion for the diagnosis (4).

A. Pratique inadaptée, persistante et répétée du jeu d'argent conduisant à une altération du fonctionnement ou une souffrance, cliniquement significative, comme en témoigne, chez le sujet, la présence d'au moins quatre des manifestations suivantes au cours d'une période de 12 mois.

1) Besoin de jouer avec des sommes d'argent croissantes pour obtenir l'état d'excitation désiré
2) Agitation ou irritabilité lors des tentatives de réduction ou d'arrêt de la pratique du jeu
3) Efforts répétés mais infructueux pour contrôler, réduire ou arrêter la pratique du jeu
4) Préoccupation par le jeu (remémoration d'expériences de jeu passées ou par la prévision de tentatives prochaines ou par des moyens de se procurer de l'argent pour jouer).
5) Joue souvent lors des sentiments de souffrance/mal être (par exemple sentiments d'impuissance, de culpabilité, d'anxiété, de dépression)
6) Après avoir perdu de l'argent au jeu, retourne souvent jouer un autre jour pour recouvrer ses pertes (pour « se refaire »)
7) Ment pour dissimuler l'ampleur réelle de ses habitudes de jeu
8) Met en danger ou a perdu une relation affective importante, un emploi ou des possibilités d'étude ou de carrière à cause du jeu
9) Compte sur les autres pour obtenir de l'argent et se sortir de situations financières désespérées dues au jeu.

B. La pratique du jeu d'argent n'est pas mieux expliquée par un épisode maniaque

Figure 1: DSM-5 criteria for pathological gambling

This reclassification from the "Impulse control disorders not elsewhere classified" section of DSM-4 to the "Substance-related and addictive disorders" section was motivated by a range of arguments suggesting a common aetiology addiction to substances (drugs, alcohol, nicotine).

(7). The diagnostic criteria in both cases include the existence of symptoms of tolerance, craving and withdrawal, as well as a feeling of loss of control and negative repercussions on various areas of personal life. In addition, a fairly strong comorbidity between pathological gambling and substance addiction has been observed (10,11), probably linked to a partially shared genetic vulnerability (12,13). In addition, certain personality traits marked by risk-seeking and impulsivity are shared gambling and substance addiction (7). This reconceptualisation of pathological gambling as addiction has implications for which consists of :

-Offering the opportunity to explore neurobiological hypotheses from the field of neurobiology. substance addiction

To open up the prospect of a "drug-free addiction" model, making it possible to study the brain mechanisms addiction without the confounding effects associated with the biochemical action of drugs. Given that the French language does not have a word specifically designating games of chance and gambling such as the term "gambling" in English, we will use the term "jeu" in our work to designate games of chance and gambling.

II. The neural circuits involved :

The neural circuits involved in pathological gambling were better explored with the advent of functional magnetic resonance imaging (fMRI) in the late 1990s (7). Neuroimaging studies have revealed structural alterations in certain brain regions in pathological gamblers. Alterations have been observed in the fronto-striatal and limbic regions of the brain, including the striatum, orbitofrontal cortex, anterior cingulate cortex, insula, hippocampus and amygdala (Figure 2). These regions are involved in impulse control, decision-making, reward processing and memory, suggesting dysfunctions in these processes in individuals affected by pathological gambling.

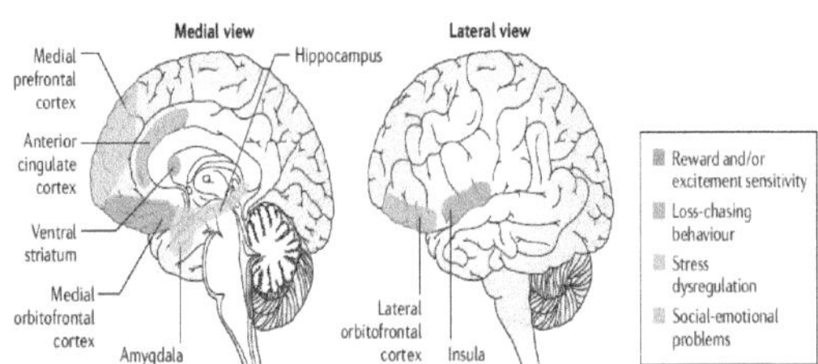

Figure 2: Brain regions involved in pathological gambling

1. Striatum

The striatum plays a crucial role in reward processing, motivation, associative learning and impulse control, making it a key brain region involved in pathological gambling. It is divided into (14): -Ventral striatum (mainly comprises the nucleus accumbens and the ventral part of the putamen) is associated with emotional regulation, motivation and associative learning (stimulus-outcome associations such as the link gambling cues and monetary gains).

- The dorsal striatum (comprising mainly the dorsal part of the putamen and the caudate nucleus) is involved in the control of voluntary movements, motor learning (stimulus-action associations, such as the link between play signals and behaviours directed towards them), habit formation and the processing of sensory and spatial information. The dorsal striatum is also involved in decision-making and impulse control.

Neuroimaging studies have shown divergent results regarding the activity of the ventral striatum in individuals suffering from pathological gambling. Some studies suggest hyperactivation, while others suggest hypoactivation or complex modulation of this brain region (15). A meta-analysis of studies on reward processing showed a relatively decreased activation of the ventral striatum during reward anticipation in individuals suffering from pathological gambling (16). This hypoactivation may suggest an alteration in reward processing or a reduction in sensitivity to reward stimuli in pathological gamblers. It may also be associated with difficulties in the reward system, such as reduced tolerance to rewards or compulsive search for higher rewards. However, preliminary studies have demonstrated larger volumes of ventral striatum (17) and increased functional connectivity of the ventral striatum. (18) in pathological gamblers compared with controls. This hyperactivation may reflect increased sensitivity to the rewards and stimuli associated with gambling, thus contributing to motivation to gamble and reward-seeking behaviour. Other preliminary studies have demonstrated associations between dopamine receptor availability in the striatum and impulsivity (such as making impulsive choices under stress) and between dopamine receptor availability in the ventral striatum and behavioural disinhibition (such as overspending) in pathological gamblers compared with healthy comparators (19,20). These results suggest that abnormalities in the ventral striatum may contribute to impulsive behaviour in these subjects. Furthermore, increased dopamine transmission in the dorsal striatum has been associated with the severity of problem gambling (21). In addition, increased binding to dopamine receptors and activation of the substantia nigra (which projects to the dorsal striatum) evoked by gambling were positively associated with the severity of problem gambling (22,23). These results suggest that increased sensitivity of the dopaminergic response in the dorsal striatum may contribute to individual variation in the severity of pathological gambling. The results of PET (positron emission tomography) scans in people with pathological gambling diverge from the reduction in striatal dopaminergic receptors reported in people with substance addictions (24,25), suggesting that the latter may represent the neurotoxic effects of substances, rather than being a mechanism of addiction.

2. Fronto-striatal circuits

The striatum projects to regions of the prefrontal cortex (PFC), in particular the medial PFC, which is involved reward-based decision-making (26).

Neuroimaging studies in pathological gambling have shown relatively decreased activity in frontostriatal regions during cue exposure (27), simulated gambling (28), inhibitory control (29) and reward anticipation (30). In addition, reduced connectivity between the striatum and medial prefrontal cortex has been implicated in cue-induced desire in pathological gambling (31).

The medial orbitofrontal cortex (involved in the subjective value of choices) and the anterior cingulate cortex (involved in the encoding of choice predictions and prediction errors) may contribute to this disorder (32). The medial orbitofrontal cortex and anterior cingulate cortex showed increased activation in response to gambling cues in people with pathological gambling, and these regions and the striatum showed reduced activation in response to gambling-related gains (33). These data suggest that regions involved in reward evaluation may be more sensitive to external cues indicating the availability of gambling than to the actual value gained or lost from gambling in pathological gamblers.

3. Insula

The insula has been implicated in interoception (34). Ventral-anterior regions are involved in the perception of bodily feedback and emotional experiences, while dorso-anterior regions are involved in higher-order cognition (35). During experimental play tasks, the insula may be involved in monitoring changes in bodily responses (such as heart rate) and encoding this information in terms of risk or arousal (36). In addition, the insula has been implicated in the cognitive evaluation of this feedback, as specific lesions of the insula can abolish cognitive distortions related to gambling, such as gambler's fallacy (defined as a mistaken belief that past events influence the probabilities of future events in a game of chance) and near-miss effect.

(37). Pathological gamblers have greater activation of the insula during cue-induced craving (38) compared to healthy individuals, In addition, people with gambling problems may have increased activation of the insula and striatum when making risk-related decisions and experiencing losses or near misses and may demonstrate increased connectivity between the insula and amygdala during these types of processes.

(39). Thus, the insula could interact abnormally with the regions involved in learning rewards and punishments in pathological gambling, which could lead to bodily feedback (such as an increase in heartbeat sensations before gambling) in the form of reward, excitement or stress signals (40).

4. Hippocampus and amygdala

The hippocampus and amygdala have been implicated emotional learning and stress regulation (41). In experimental gaming tasks, the hippocampus has been implicated in probabilistic learning of stimulus-outcome contingencies. (for example, predicting when gambling cues indicate rewards versus punishments) and the amygdala has been implicated in loss aversion-oriented cost-benefit analyses (42). In real-world gambling, probabilistic learning may be challenged by intermittent reward programmes in gambling devices such as electronic gaming machines, suggesting that playing certain forms of gambling may influence decision-making tendencies (43).

III. The reward system and game phases

Studies have looked at the cerebral processing of reward in the different phases of play. As has already been documented, the **"reward system"** mainly ncludes the striatum, ventromedial prefrontal cortex, orbitofrontal cortex and amygdala (Figure 3).

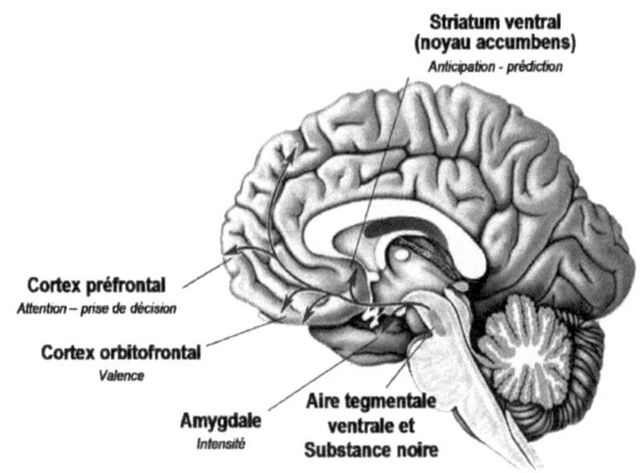

Figure 3: The reward system

The first fMRI studies focused on the **"reward reception"** phase. This phase concerns the sensitivity of pathological gamblers to monetary gains and losses in the context of gambling or gambling addiction. learning process. The results of these studies highlighted a hypoactivation of the reward system in response to monetary gains in gamblers, particularly in the ventral striatum and prefrontal cortex (28,29) (Figure 4). According to one of these studies, the severity of pathological gambling symptoms was even correlated with the intensity of this hypoactivation (28). This result refers to the theoretical framework of the **"reward deficiency syndrome"**, which considers addiction to be the consequence of chronic hypo-sensitivity to reward.

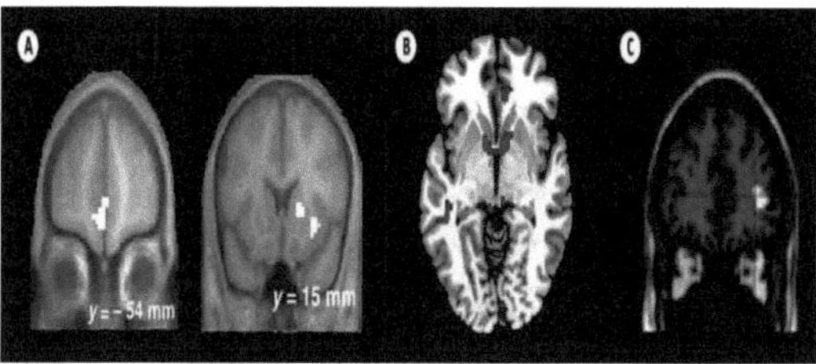

Figure 4: Hypoactivation of the reward system in response to monetary gains in pathological gamblers

However, other more recent studies have not found the same thing, and have instead shown signs hypersensitivity to reward in pathological gamblers. In a study by Miedl et al, a fronto-parietal cortical circuit was hyperactivated by directly comparing wins and losses in a blackjack game (44). Similarly, two electroencephalography experiments showed a clear amplification neuronal activity from the medial prefrontal cortex in response to monetary winnings in gamblers (45,46).With regard to the **"reward anticipation"** phase, which corresponds to the phase of expectation and uncertainty in gambling, the results were also mixed. An initial study showed a reactivity decreased reactivity of the reward system in gamblers (47). In contrast, a second study showed increased reactivity in the dorsal striatum anticipating large monetary gains (48). These inconsistencies between the different studies, which are reminiscent of those observed substance addiction (49), are currently the subject of intense debate (50). Recently, a study by Sescousse et al (7) proposed the hypothesis that the relevant process to study was not sensitivity to monetary rewards, but rather sensitivity to non-monetary rewards. In fact, the case of chronic hypersensitivity to non-monetary rewards (such sex, food, etc.), the motivation for monetary rewards would automatically take over and eventually lead to behaviour geared almost exclusively towards . To test this hypothesis, Secousse et al. compared brain responses to stimuli predicting monetary gains or erotic images (Figure 5). The results of this experiment concluded that healthy subjects showed similar cerebral responses in the striatum for the two types of reward, whereas pathological gamblers showed a clear decrease in reactivity for stimuli predicting erotic images compared with those predicting monetary gains (51). This difference in reactivity, which was found to correlate with the severity of gambling symptoms, could be a key marker of gambling addiction.

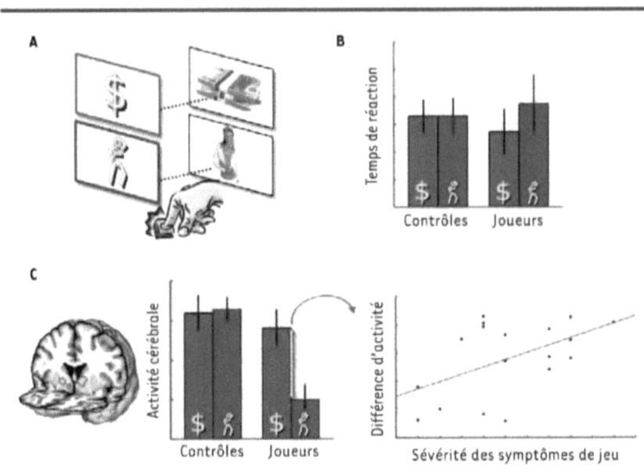

Figure 5: Reduced reactivity when anticipating non money in pathological gamblers

In relation to sensitivity to gains and losses, several studies have suggested dysfunctions in learning mechanisms and **"prediction errors",** which refer to the inaccuracies or false anticipations that gamblers make when predicting the outcome of gambling-related events. These are surprise signals that reflect the difference between the perceived value and the expected or predicted value of the rewards. These signals are emitted by the midbrain and are then transmitted to the striatum (52). They play a vital role in learning the predicted value of rewards. If the expected value is lower than the perceived value, the prediction error is positive and helps to increase the expected value in the future. On the other hand, if the expected value is greater than perceived value, the prediction error is negative and contributes to reducing the expected value in the future (52). The mechanisms prediction have been studied by Voon et al (53) in a reinforcement learning task in Parkinson's patients who had developed addictive behaviours following dopaminergic treatment. The results showed the potentiating effect of dopamine in these patients, as evidenced by an amplification of the positive prediction error signal from the ventral striatum. This mechanism may explain a biased sensitivity in favour of rewards, and therefore of addictive behaviour. Other research has looked at the **"near-miss"** effect the context . This is the feeling you get when you lose and you were very close to winning. For example, in a slot machine, if the symbols lined up are almost all the same, but not quite, this creates the illusion of almost winning, even though the player has technically lost. In normal subjects, near-miss events increase the desire to continue gambling and activate the reward system (particularly the striatum), possibly reflecting the calculation of a positive prediction error (54). However, in pathological gamblers, researchers have observed a correlation between the midbrain response to near-miss events and the severity of gambling symptoms (55). This finding suggests that the cognitive and neurophysiological distortion associated with near-miss events could be a marker of gambling addiction. In line with the numerous fMRI studies conducted on substance addiction, some experiments have investigated **the reactivity of pathological gamblers to environmental cues predictive of gambling**. In a first study, Potenza et al (54) used videos of actors emotionally describing their casino gambling experience. The results showed that the desire to gamble (craving) aroused by these videos was associated with a reduction activity in the ventromedial prefrontal cortex, striatum and thalamus of pathological gamblers. This result is surprising, given that the majority of Studies on substance addiction have reported hyperactivation in these same regions (56,57). However, it should be noted that the interpretation of these results was relatively delicate due to the complexity of the videos used, which presented gambling cues indirectly through the description of an actor. In contrast to this first study, two other experiments found cerebral hyperactivations in pathological gamblers viewing photos or videos illustrating gambling scenes in casinos (58,59). In both cases, the hyperactivated regions included the dorsolateral prefrontal cortex, the parahippocampal gyrus and the occipital cortex, while the study by Goudriaan et al. also reported hyperactivation of the posterior cingulate cortex and the amygdala. Given the involvement of these regions in memory, emotional and visual processes, the authors concluded that gambling cues have an exacerbated salience in pathological gamblers. Finally, two looked at the **risk assessment** phase of a blackjack game (16,32). The results showed an increase in activity in the striatum and orbitofrontal cortex of pathological gamblers in high-risk trials compared with low-risk trials. According to the authors, this result reflects high level of excitement experienced by gamblers in high-risk situations, and therefore the high addictive potential of these situations.Neuroimaging studies on pathological gambling are still few and far between, and it is not yet possible to construct a coherent neurobiological model of pathological gambling. Nevertheless, two conclusions can be drawn. Firstly, pathological gamblers appear to show hypoactivation of the ventromedial prefrontal cortex in response to monetary gains. In addition, the presentation of environmental cues related to gambling seems to generate cerebral hyperactivations, probably reflecting hyperreactivity to stimuli conditioned by gambling. This phenomenon could be exacerbated by hyposensitivity to non-monetary rewards, which in contrast increases the motivational salience of monetary rewards.

IV.Structural alterations to the brain

To date, only a few studies have focused on structural changes in the brain in pathological gambling and have reported mixed results. Some magnetic resonance imaging (MRI) studies aimed at identifying grey matter abnormalities have not revealed significant volumetric differences between subjects diagnosed with gambling disorder and healthy individuals (61-63). However, other studies have reported significant thinning of grey matter in prefrontal regions (64,65). In addition, a decrease in the volumes of the hippocampus and amygdala has been demonstrated (66,67). MRI studies using diffusion tensor imaging to white matter integrity have instead detected a fairly consistent reduction in white matter integrity in pathological gamblers (61), even without grey matter abnormalities (68)raising the question of a possible pre-existing vulnerability to the progressive neuroadaptive changes induced by sustained gambling.

V. Role of neurotransmitters

1. Dopamine

A. Neurochemical studies :

Several studies substance addiction have highlighted the central role of dopamine. This neuromodulator, abundant in subcortical structures such as the striatum, is involved in reward and reinforcement processes. It is released in large quantities by most psychoactive substances (69). In the 2000s, a series of studies using Positron Emission Tomography (PET) showed a reduction in the density of D2 dopamine receptors in the striatum of individuals addicted to cocaine, heroin, methamphetamine or alcohol (69) (Figure 6).This result has been interpreted in the framework of **the hypodopaminergic theory** of addiction.This theory states that under-stimulation of the dopaminergic system would reduce sensitivity to rewards (hence the name of the theory: "**reward deficiency syndrome**"), and would lead to excessive drug use in order to compensate for this deficit (70). However, recent PET studies of pathological gamblers have failed to validate this hypothesis in the case of pathological gambling (23,61). Thus, although two of these studies showed an inverse correlation between the severity of gambling symptoms and D2 receptor density, neither study was able to show a systematic reduction compared with control subjects (21) (Figure 6).

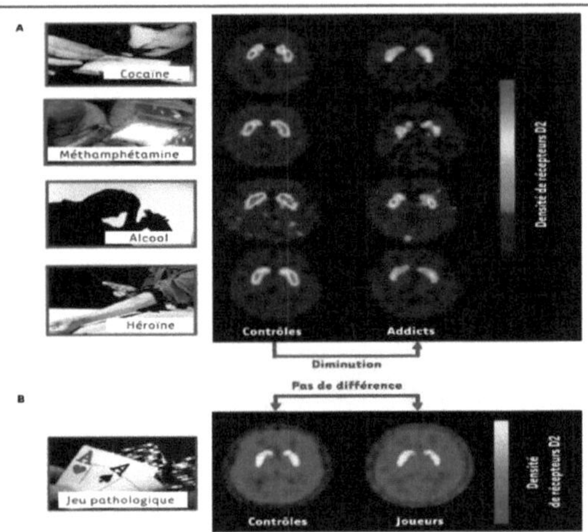

Figure 6: PET mapping of D2 dopamine receptors in the striatum

Similarly, the few pharmacological studies conducted to date have produced heterogeneous results. In their first study, Zack and Poulos looked at the effects of amphetamines (dopamine agonists) on the behaviour of pathological gamblers, based on the observation that the administration of a small dose of amphetamines to drug addicts seems to play a motivational role. Their results confirmed this prediction, showing an increase in the desire to gamble and in the speed of reading gambling-related words. (71). Unexpectedly, however, the same effects were observed a second study in which the players were given haloperidol, a selective D2 dopamine receptor antagonist (72). One possible explanation for this apparent contradiction lies in the hypothesis that a low dose of dopamine antagonist could act on inhibitory presynaptic auto-receptors, thereby increasing dopamine transmission (39). Although these studies confirm the primordial role of dopamine in gambling behaviour, unfortunately they do not provide any answers as to the direction of this effect in pathological gambling.

B. Genetic studies

At the same time, a number of studies have looked at genetic variations thought to affect dopaminergic function in the brain. These studies have focused on the DRD2 gene coding for D2 receptors, and in particular on the Taq1A polymorphism, which influences the density of D2 receptors in the brain and has been associated with substance addiction (69). An initial study showed an association between this polymorphism and pathological gambling, suggesting a reduction in the concentration of D2 receptors and therefore the hypodopaminergic hypothesis (72). However, this result should be treated with caution, insofar as it was not reproduced in a more recent study and the association of the Taq1A polymorphism with The link between the DRD2 gene and the regulation of D2 dopamine receptors has been called into question (19). Other associations have nevertheless been shown between pathological gambling and the DRD4 (23,45) and DRD1 (21,72) genes, confirming the likely involvement of dopamine in the dysregulation of gambling behaviour.

C. Parkinson's disease and pathological gambling

Another strong argument in favour of this hypothesis comes from repeated clinical observations showing the appearance of addictive behaviour in a number of Parkinson's patients. These patients, who suffer from degeneration of the dopaminergic neurons in the substantia nigra and in particular from motor disorders, are generally treated with dopaminergic agonists. However, it has been observed that this treatment leads to symptoms of pathological gambling, as well as hypersexuality, compulsive buying and bulimia (73). The incidence of pathological gambling in these patients is of the order of , compared with 1 to 2% in the general population, and seems to be more closely linked to treatment with dopaminergic agonists, which have a strong affinity for the D3 receptors present in large quantities in the ventral striatum (74). Although the nature of the interaction between Parkinson's disease and the mechanism of action of dopamine agonists remains to be elucidated, these empirical observations highlight the role of dopamine in the development of pathological gambling. One of the hypotheses put forward suggests that treatment with agonists, designed essentially to restore dopaminergic function in the dorsal striatum - which specialises in motor functions - could cause an overdose of dopamine in the ventral striatum - which specialises in motivational functions and is relatively spared in Parkinson's disease (39). This mechanism, which could explain the compulsive behaviour of certain patients,therefore point to a hyperdopaminergic view addiction, contrast to the 'reward' theory deficiency syndrome". Overall, these data confirm the existence of a probable dysregulation of dopaminergic function in pathological gambling, but remain too heterogeneous to draw clear and precise conclusions as to the mechanisms involved.

2. Noradrenaline

Norepinephrine is a catecholamine structurally related epinephrine that is released in response to stress and affects the sympathetic nervous system response. Norepinephrine can be synthesised from dopamine and can have systemic (central and peripheral) effects (75). The noradrenergic system, which uses norepinephrine as its main chemical messenger, is responsible for several brain functions, including wakefulness, attention, mood, learning, memory and response to stress (76). In preclinical models of substance dependence, norepinephrine is critically involved in mediating stimulant effects, including sensitisation and reinstatement of drug seeking (77).

Similar to substance dependence, behavioural addiction also involves an arousal linked to norepinephrine, which can mimic a sensation of 'pleasure'. Norepinephrine has been studied in pathological gambling since the 1980s. Activation of the sympathetic system, marked by an increase in heart rate and changes in other physical parameters, is present in gamblers and appears to be more pronounced in pathological gamblers (78). In addition, studies have found higher concentrations of noradrenaline or its metabolites in the blood, urine and cerebrospinal fluid of pathological gamblers compared with a control population (78). Noradrenaline therefore seems to play an important role stimulation and excitement during gambling situations. In addition Individuals with gambling disorders maintained significantly higher noradrenergic levels throughout a gambling session, whereas healthy controls showed elevated levels only at the beginning of the gambling session (79). Noradrenergic function has been linked to sensation-seeking behaviour in gambling disorders, which shares some similarities with substance dependence. Overactivity of the noradrenergic system in gambling disorders may reinforce and/or maintain gambling behaviour through influences on arousal (80). Furthermore, it has been shown that adrenergic drugs can influence specific aspects of impulse control in animal and human studies. These findings suggest several possible roles for adrenergic function in pathological gambling and its treatment, and further research is needed in this area to examine these possibilities (9).

3. Serotonin

Serotonin is also a neurotransmitter involved in the control of impulsivity. Abnormal serotonin function has been associated with poor impulse control. Neurochemical studies suggest serotonin similarities in non-substance and substance addiction (81). Pathological gamblers, like other subjects with impulse control disorders, show a decrease in the concentration of the serotonin metabolite5-hydroxyindoleacetic acid, in cerebrospinal fluid compared with control subjects (78). In another study, the density of the platelet serotonin transporter (SERT), a protein that regulates the synaptic concentration of serotonin by reuptake mechanisms, was decreased in pathological gamblers, suggesting the involvement of serotonin in gambling disorder (82). Administration of meta-chlorophenyl piperazine (m-CPP), a serotonergic agonist, produces a euphoric effect in pathological gamblers. This effect is observed other populations of patients substance-related addiction, but not in control populations (78).

4. Opioids :

The opioid system consists of several types of receptors (μ, δ and κ) and peptides (β-endorphin, enkephalins and dynorphins). Ligands of μ and δ opioid receptors can produce rewarding effects, while ligands of κ opioid receptors can have aversive effects (83). Preclinical evidence indicates that opioid receptors are widely distributed in the mesolimbic system and are involved in hedonic aspects of reward processing (84). Opioid function can modify dopamine release in the mesolimbic pathway extending from the ventral tegmental area to the nucleus accumbens or ventral striatum and influence the pleasure experienced during addictive behaviour (85). Thus, individuals with an altered opiate system experience intense euphoria and consequently have greater difficulty controlling behaviours linked to the addictive object.

Gambling has been associated with elevated blood levels of the endogenous β-opioid endorphin and modulation of the opioid system by opioid receptor antagonists and partial agonists has shown significant promise in the treatment of gambling disorder. An fMRI study of the opioid antagonist μ

"In a multicentre trial of the opioid antagonist naloxone, attenuated reward-related responses in the ventral striatum and enhanced loss-related activity in the medial prefrontal cortex were observed during a wheel of fortune task in healthy volunteers (86). In a multicentre trial of the opioid antagonist nalmefene in the treatment of gambling disorder, participants who received this agent showed a statistically significant reduction in the severity of gambling disorder (87). Similarly subjects who reported strong gambling urges at the start of treatment responded better to naltrexone than to placebo (88).

5. Glutamate :

A persuasive body of preclinical evidence has indicated a role for glutamate, the most abundant excitatory neurotransmitter, in drug-related reward, reinforcement and relapse (89). Glutamate appears to be involved in long-lasting neuroadaptations in the corticostriatal brain circuit. It has also been shown that imbalances in glutamate homeostasis lead to changes in neuroplasticity, altering communication between the prefrontal cortex and the nucleus accumbens and resulting in reward-seeking behaviour (90). Data from cerebrospinal fluid studies also suggest a dysfunctional glutamate system in pathological gamblers (90). In parallel with substance dependence, N-acetyl cysteine (NAC) has been shown to significantly reduce the severity of pathological gambling. In addition, open-label administration of memantine, an N-methyl-D-aspartate receptor antagonist, has shown promise in reducing the severity of pathological gambling and cognitive inflexibility in gambling disorder (91).

VI. Therapeutic implications :

Knowing which regions of the brain and which neurotransmitters are involved in pathological gambling can point the way towards pharmacological therapeutic strategies. At present, no drug has received regulatory approval for the treatment of gambling disorders. However, a number of double-blind, placebo-controlled trials of various pharmacological agents have demonstrated the superiority of active drugs over placebo in the treatment of gambling disorders, although this effectiveness remains mixed from one study to another (80).

1. Opioid receptor antagonists

Opioid receptor antagonists, such as naltrexone or nalmefene, are the class of drugs that has probably received the most attention for the treatment of gambling disorder (92), given their ability to modulate dopaminergic transmission in the mesolimbic pathway. Four double-blind, placebo-controlled studies have supported the efficacy of opioid receptor antagonists to varying degrees. A 12-week placebo-controlled trial with naltrexone demonstrated a reduction in gambling urges and behaviours in 45 people with gambling disorder compared with placebo. These results were confirmed in a second study of 77 people over a period of 18 weeks (93). In addition, two multicentre, placebo-controlled studies have demonstrated the efficacy of nalmefene (which has a lower risk of hepatotoxicity than naltrexone) in the treatment of gambling disorder. In the first study involving 207 people, 59% of participants who received nalmefene for 16 weeks showed significant reductions in gambling urges, thoughts and behaviours, compared with only 34% of participants who received a placebo (74). In the second study, primary and secondary outcomes in the intention-to-treat population were not significantly different with nalmefene compared with placebo, but post-hoc analyses of participants who received full titration of nalmefene for at least 1 week showed a significantly greater reduction in the primary outcome measure compared with placebo (94). Finally, a pooled analysis of 284 participants in two of these studies showed that a positive response to either nalmefene or naltrexone was significantly associated with a positive family history of alcoholism, and that the intensity of gambling cravings in an individual was associated with a positive response at higher doses (74).

2. The antidepressants

Early models of pathological gambling and gambling disorder suggested a role for serotonin, particularly in impulse control. Selective serotonin reuptake inhibitors (SSRIs) were one of the first drugs used to treat gambling disorders. Controlled clinical trials evaluating SSRIs have shown mixed results for behavioural addictions (92). Five double-blind, placebo-controlled pharmacological studies of serotonin reuptake inhibitors for gambling disorder have been conducted. Although the initial studies of fluvoxamine and paroxetine demonstrated some benefit over placebo (95,96), subsequent studies of fluvoxamine, paroxetine and sertraline failed to separate these effects from those of placebo (92,97). SSRI treatments remain an active area of investigation and further research is required to assess the potential clinical use SSRIs for gambling disorders and other behavioural addictions.

3. antipsychotics

Given the roles of the dopaminergic and serotonergic systems gambling disorder, two studies have examined the efficacy of olanzapine, a dopamine and serotonin receptor antagonist, in the treatment of gambling disorder, but neither study demonstrated superiority of olanzapine over placebo(98).

4. Glutamatergic agents :

Given the preliminary human data suggesting a dysfunctional glutamatergic system in gambling disorder, N-acetylcysteine (NAC), a glutamate-modulating agent that appears to be useful in treating people with substance-related disorders, was administered to 27 adults with gambling disorder, with responders then receiving a double-blind trial blinded to a further 6 weeks of NAC or placebo. In the open-label phase, 59% of participants experienced significant reductions in gambling symptoms, and at the end of the double-blind phase, 83% of those receiving NAC were still classified as responders, compared with 29% of receiving placebo. A controlled, double-blind, 12-week follow-up study combining NAC with CBT including elements of motivational interviewing and imaginal desensitisation in 28 people also addicted to nicotine demonstrated a significant benefit with NAC treatment compared with placebo on nicotine dependence symptoms during treatment, and on problem gambling symptoms 3 months after the end of formal treatment (99).

On the basis of these neurobiological foundations of pathological gambling and effective pharmacotherapies for drug addiction and other psychiatric disorders Bullock et al. proposed this algorithm for the pharmacological treatment of this disorder (100) (Figure 7).

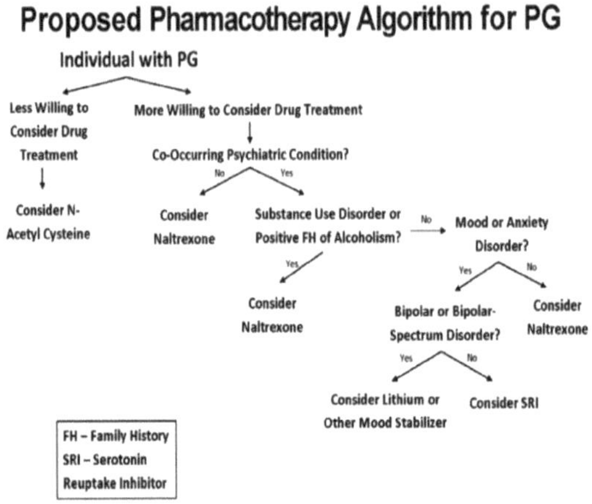

Figure 7: Algorithm for the treatment of pathological gambling

CONCLUSION

Gambling is a recreational activity for most people. However, some gamblers lose control and gamble excessively, with dramatic financial, personal and professional consequences. The many similarities with substance addiction have led the psychiatric community to redefine pathological gambling as a behavioural addiction, currently recognised as such in the fifth version of the Diagnostic and Statistical Manual of Mental Disorders (DSM- 5). Gambling disorder is now a public health problem, with an estimated prevalence of 1 to 2% in Western countries. Over the last decade, considerable progress has been made in understanding the neurobiological basis of this disorder, particularly with the advent of neuroimaging. Hence the interest of our work, which aims to better illustrate the neurobiological basis of pathological gambling. Several neurotransmitter systems (norepinephrine, serotonin, dopamine, opioids and glutamate) and brain regions (ventral striatum, ventromedial prefrontal cortex, insula) have been implicated. A better understanding of the neurobiological mechanisms of pathological gambling therefore seems important for developing more targeted prevention and treatment strategies.To meet our objective, a systematic review of the literature was carried out using the Prisma-P methodology. Bibliographic references were managed using Zotero software. The search queries were entered into Pubmed using the following terms: "Neurobiology", "Gambling Disorder", "Pathological Gambling", "Gambling", etc. The search was conducted from 1997 to 2024 and identified 208 references. After excluding duplicates, 202 references were retained. The inclusion criteria were clinical trials, randomised controlled trials and systematic reviews published from 1997 to 2024 with the primary or secondary objective of studying the various neurobiological mechanisms of pathological gambling. Only 27 items met our criteria and were included in our search. Following these procedures, a Prisma flow chart was drawn up. According to the literature, the main neurobiological mechanisms of pathological gambling are :

-dysfunction of the cerebral circuits of the "reward system, particularly in the striatum and ventromedial prefrontal cortex

-dysfunction of the dopaminergic system (dopamine and dopamine receptors)

-Involvement of other noradrenergic, serotonergic, glutamatergic and opoid systems, with preliminary evidence of the efficacy of drugs which modify these neurotransmitters.

However, the studies carried out to date are still too few and heterogeneous to build a coherent neurobiological model of pathological gambling, and many grey areas remain. Replication of results and diversification of research approaches will be necessary in the coming years in order to consolidate the current model. The development of animal models of pathological gambling is a particularly interesting avenue, facilitating the use of pharmacological manipulations and longitudinal studies.

REFERENCES

1. Potenza MN. Should addictive disorders include non-substance-related conditions? Addiction. Sept 2006;101 Suppl 1:142-51.

2. Raylu N, Oei TP. Role of culture in gambling and problem gambling. Clin Psychol Rev 23:1087-114.

3. Potenza MN, Balodis IM, Derevensky J, Grant JE, Petry NM, Verdejo-Garcia A, et al. Gambling disorder. Nat Rev Dis Primers. 25 Jul 2019;5(1):1-21.

4. American Psychiatric Association. Diagnostic and Statistical Manual of Mental Disorders 5th ed. Washington, DC: American Psychiatric Association, 2013.

5. Welte JW, Barnes GM, Tidwell MC, et al. Gambling and problem gambling in the United States: changes between 1999 and 2013. J Gambl Stud 2014; doi: 10.1007/s10899-014- 9471-4.

6. Potenza MN, Balodis IM, Derevensky J, Grant JE, Petry NM, Verdejo-Garcia A, et al. Gambling disorder. Nat Rev Dis Primers. 25 Jul 2019;5(1):51.

7. Sescousse G. Addiction aux jeux d'argent - Apport des neurosciences et de la neuro-imagerie. Med Sci (Paris). 1 August 2015;31(8-9):784-91.

8. Potenza MN. Neurobiology of gambling behaviors. Curr Opin Neurobiol. August 2013;23(4):660-7.

9. Potenza MN. Review. The neurobiology of pathological gambling and drug addiction: an overview and new findings. Philos Trans R Soc Lond B Biol Sci. 12 Oct 2008;363(1507):3181-9.

10. Goudriaan AE, Oosterlaan J, de Beurs E, Van den Brink W. Pathological gambling: a comprehensive review of biobehavioral findings. Neurosci

Biobehav Rev 2004; 28: 123- 141.

11. Petry NM, Stinson FS, Grant BF. Comorbidity of DSM-IV pathological gambling and other psychiatric disorders: results from the National epidemiologic survey on alcohol and
related conditions. J Clin Psychiatry 2005; 66: 564-574.

12. Eisen SA, Slutskte WS, Lyons MJ, et al. The genetics of pathological gambling. Semin Clin Neuropsychiatry 2001; 6: 195-204.

13. Slutske WS, Eisen S, True WR, et al. Common genetic vulnerability for pathological gambling and alcohol dependence in men. Arch Gen Psychiatry 2000; 57: 666-673.

14. Jessup, R. K. & O'Doherty, J. P. Human dorsal striatal activity during choice discriminates reinforcement learning behavior from the gambler's fallacy. J. Neurosci. 31, 6296-6304 (2011).

15. Clark, L., Boileau, I. & Zack, M. Neuroimaging of reward mechanisms in gambling disorder: an integrative review. Mol. Psychiatry 24, 674-693 (2018).

16. Machielse, M. W. J. & Sescousse, G. Disruption of reward processing in addiction: an image- based meta-analysis of functional magnetic resonance imaging studies. JAMA Psychiatry 74, 387-398 (2017). This work is a meta-analysis showing similarities and differences in the neural correlates of reward processing in individuals with gambling and SUDs.

17. Koehler, S., Hasselmann, E., Wustenberg, T., Heinz, A. & Romanczuk-Seiferth, N. Higher volume of ventral striatum and right prefrontal cortex in pathological gambling. Brain Struct. Funct. 220, 469-477 (2015).

18. Contreras- Rodriguez, O. et al. Cocaine- specific neuroplasticity in the ventral striatum network are linked to delay discounting and drug relapse. Addiction 110, 1953-1962 (2015).

19. Clark, L. et al. Striatal dopamine D2/D3 receptor binding in pathological gambling is correlated with mood- related impulsivity. Neuroimage 63, 40-46 (2012).

20. Lawrence, A. D., Brooks, D. J. & Whone, A. L. Ventral striatal dopamine synthesis capacity predicts financial extravagance in Parkinson's disease. Front. Psychol. 4, 90 (2013).

21. Boileau, I. et al. In vivo evidence for greater amphetamine-induced dopamine release in pathological gambling: a positron emission tomography study with [11C]-(+)-PHNO. Mol. Psychiatry 19, 1305-1313 (2014).

22. Chase, H. W. & Clark, L. Gambling severity predicts midbrain response to near- miss outcomes. J. Neurosci. 30, 6180-6187 (2010).

23. Boileau, I. et al. The D2/3 dopamine receptor in pathological gambling: a positron emission tomography study with [11C]-(+)-propylhexahydro- naphtho-oxazin and [11C]raclopride. Addiction 108, 953-963 (2013).

24. Volkow, N. D. et al. Decreased striatal dopaminergic responsiveness in detoxified cocaine-dependent subjects. Nature 386, 830-833 (1997).

25. Heinz, A. et al. Correlation between dopamine D2 receptors in the ventral striatum and central processing of alcohol cues and craving. Am. J. Psychiatry 161, 1783-1789 (2004).

26. Allain, F., Minogianis, E. A., Roberts, D. C. & Samaha, A. N. How fast and how often: the pharmacokinetics of drug use are decisive in addiction. Neurosci. Biobehav. Rev. 56,166-179 (2015).

27. Potenza, M. N. et al. Gambling urges in pathological gambling: a functional magnetic resonance imaging study. Arch. Gen. Psychiatry 60, 828-836 (2003).

28. Reuter J, Raedler T, Rose M, et al. Pathological gambling is linked to

reduced activation of the mesolimbic reward system. Nat Neurosci 2005; 8: 147-148.

29. De Ruiter MB, Veltman DJ, Goudriaan AE, et al. Response perseveration and ventral
prefrontal sensitivity to reward and punishment in male problem gamblers and smokers. Neuropsychopharmacology 2009; 34: 1027-1038.

30. Balodis IM, Kober H, Worhunsky PD, et al. Diminished frontostriatal activity during processing of monetary rewards and losses in pathological gambling. Biol Psychiatry 2012; 71: 749-757.

31. Limbrick- Oldfield, E. H. et al. Neural substrates of cue reactivity and craving in gambling disorder. Transl Psychiatry 7, e992 (2017).

32. Kennerley, S. W., Behrens, T. E. & Wallis, J. D. Double dissociation of value computations in orbitofrontal and anterior cingulate neurons. Nat. Neurosci. 14, 1581-1589 (2011).

33. Wallis, J. D. & Kennerley, S. W. Contrasting reward signals in the orbitofrontal cortex and anterior cingulate cortex. Ann. NY Acad. Sci. 1239, 33-42 (2011).

34. Craig, A. D. How do you feel - now? The anterior insula and human awareness. Nat. Rev. Neurosci. 10, 59-70 (2009).

35. Droutman, V., Read, S. J. & Bechara, A. Revisiting the role of the insula in addiction. Trends Cogn. Sci. 19, 414-420 (2015).

36. Panitz, C., Wacker, J., Stemmler, G. & Mueller, E. M. Brain-heart coupling at the P300 latency is linked to anterior cingulate cortex and insula — a cardio-electroencephalographic covariance tracing study. Biol. Psychol. 94, 185-191 (2013).

37. Potenza, M. N. The neural bases of cognitive processes in gambling

disorder. Trends Cogn. Sci. 18, 429-438 (2014).

38. Limbrick- Oldfield, E. H. et al. Neural substrates of cue reactivity and craving in gambling disorder. Transl Psychiatry 7, e992 (2017).

39. Clark, L., Lawrence, A. J., Astley- Jones, F. & Gray, N. Gambling near-misses enhance motivation to gamble and recruit win- related brain circuitry. Neuron 61, 481-490 (2009).

40. Verdejo- Garcia, A., Clark, L. & Dunn, B. D. The role of interoception in addiction: a critical review. Neurosci. Biobehav. Rev. 36, 1857-1869 (2012).

41. Dedovic, K., Duchesne, A., Andrews, J., Engert, V. & Pruessner, J. C. The brain and the stress axis: the neural correlates of cortisol regulation in response to stress. Neuroimage 47, 864-871 (2009).

42. Shohamy, D., Myers, C. E., Hopkins, R. O., Sage, J. & Gluck, M. A. Distinct hippocampal and basal ganglia contributions to probabilistic learning and reversal. J. Cogn. Neurosci. 21, 1821-1833 (2009).

43. Rahman, A. S., Xu, J. & Potenza, M. N. Hippocampal and amygdalar volumetric differences in pathological gambling: a preliminary study of the associations with the behavioral inhibition system. Neuropsychopharmacology 39, 738-745 (2014).

44. Miedl SF, Fehr T, Meyer G, Herrmann M. Neurobiological correlates of problem gambling in a quasi-realistic blackjack scenario as revealed by fMRI. Psychiatry Res. 30 March 2010;181(3):165-73.

45. Oberg SA, Christie GJ, Tata MS. Problem gamblers exhibit reward hypersensitivity in medial frontal cortex during gambling. Neuropsychologia 2011 ; 49 : 3768-3775.

46. Hewig J, Kretschmer N, Trippe RH, et al. Hypersensitivity to reward in problem gamblers. Biol Psychiatry 2010 ; 67 : 781-783.

47. Balodis IM, Potenza MN. Anticipatory reward processing in addicted populations: a focus on the monetary incentive delay task. Biol Psychiatry. March 1, 2015;77(5):434-44.

48. van den Bos R, Lasthuis W, den Heijer E, van der Harst J, Spruijt B. Toward a rodent model of the Iowa gambling task. Behav Res Methods. August 2006;38(3):470-8.

49. Hommer DW, Bjork JM, Gilman JM. Imaging brain response to reward in addictive disorders. Ann NY Acad Sci 2011; 1216: 50-61.

50. Leyton M, Vezina P. On cue: striatal ups and downs in addictions. Biol Psychiatry 2012; 72: e21.

51. Sescousse G, Barbalat G, Domenech P, Dreher JC. Imbalance in the sensitivity to different types of rewards in pathological gambling. Brain 2013; 136: 2527-2538.

52. Schultz W. Multiple reward signals in the brain. Nat Rev Neurosci 2000; 1: 199-207.

53. Voon V, Napier TC, Frank MJ, Sgambato-Faure V, Grace AA, Rodriguez-Oroz M, et al. Impulse control disorders and levodopa-induced dyskinesias in Parkinson's disease: an update. Lancet Neurol. March 2017;16(3):238-50.

54. Potenza MN, Winters KC. The neurobiology of pathological gambling: translating research findings into clinical advances. J Gambl Stud. 2003;19(1):7-10.

55. Chase HW, Clark L. Gambling severity predicts midbrain response to near-miss outcomes. J Neurosci 2010 ; 30 : 6180-6187.

56. Garavan H, Pankiewicz J, Bloom A, et al. Cue-induced cocaine craving: neuroanatomical specificity for drug users and drug stimuli. Am J Psychiatry

2000; 157: 1789-1798.

57. David SP, Munafà MR, Johansen-Berg H, et al. Ventral striatum/nucleus accumbens activation to smoking-related pictorial cues in smokers and nonsmokers: a functional magnetic resonance imaging study. Biol Psychiatry 2005 ; 58 : 488-494.

58. Goudriaan AE, de Ruiter MB, van den Brink W, et al. Brain activation patterns associated with cue reactivity and craving in abstinent problem gamblers, heavy smokers and
healthy controls: an fMRI study. Addict Biol 2010; 15: 491-503.

59. Crockford DN, Goodtear B, Edwards J, et al. Cue-induced brain activity in pathological gamblers. Biol Psychiatry 2005; 58: 787-795.

60. Power Y, Goodyear B, Crockford D. Neural correlates of pathological gamblers. preference for immediate rewards during the Iowa gambling task: an fMRI study. J Gambl Stud 2012; 28: 623-636.

61. Joutsa, J., Saunavaara, J., Parkkola, R., Niemela, S., Kaasinen, V., 2011. Extensive abnormality of brain white matter integrity in pathological gambling. Psychiatry Res. 194, 340- 346.

62. van Holst, R.J., de Ruiter, M.B., van den Brink, W., Veltman, D.J., Goudriaan, A.E., 2012a. A voxel-based morphometry study comparing problem gamblers, alcohol abusers, and healthy controls. Drug Alcohol Depend. 124, 142- 148.

63. Yip, S.W., Morie, K.P., Xu, J., Constable, R.T., Malison, R.T., Carroll, K.M., Potenza, M.N., 2017b. Shared microstructural features of behavioral and substance addictions revealed in areas of crossing fibers. Biol. Psychiatry Cogn. Neurosci. Neuroimaging. 2, 188-195.

64. Grant, J.E., Odlaug, B.L., Chamberlain, S.R., 2015. Reduced cortical

thickness in gambling disorder: a morphometric MRI study. Eur. Arch. Psychiatry Clin. Neurosci. 265, 655- 661.

65. Zois, E., Kiefer, F., Lemenager, T., Vollstadt-Klein, S., Mann, K., Fauth-Bühler, M., 2017.
Frontal cortex gray matter volume alterations in pathological gambling occur independently from substance use disorder. Addict. Biol. 22, 864- 872.

66. Fuentes, D., Rzezak, P., Pereira, F.R., Malloy-Diniz, L.F., Santos, L.C., Duran, F.L.,
Barreiros, M.A., Castro, C.C., Busatto, G.F., Tavares, H., Gorenstein, C., 2015. Mapping brain volumetric abnormalities in never-treated pathological gamblers. Psychiatry Res. 232, 208-213.

67. Rahman, A.S., Xu, J., Potenza, M.N., 2014. Hippocampal and amygdalar volumetric
differences in pathological gambling: a preliminary study of the associations with the behavioral inhibition system. Neuropsychopharmacology. 39, 738- 745.

68. Yip, S.W., Morie, K.P., Xu, J., Constable, R.T., Malison, R.T., Carroll, K.M., Potenza, M.N., 2017b. Shared microstructural features of behavioral and substance addictions revealed in areas of crossing fibers. Biol. Psychiatry Cogn. Neurosci. Neuroimaging. 2, 188-195.

69. Volkow ND, Wang GJ, Fowler JS, et al. Addiction: beyond dopamine reward circuitry. Proc Natl Acad Sci USA 2011; 108: 15037-15042.

70. Comings DE, Blum K. Reward deficiency syndrome: genetic aspects of behavioral disorders. Prog Brain Res 2000; 126: 325-341.

71. Zack M, Poulos CX. Amphetamine primes motivation to gamble and gambling-related semantic networks in problem gamblers. Neuropsychopharmacology 2004; 29: 195- 207.

72. Zack M, Poulos CX. A D2 antagonist enhances the rewarding and priming effects of a gambling episode in pathological gamblers. Neuropsychopharmacology 2007; 32: 1678- 1686.

73. Dagher A, Robbins TW. Personality, addiction, dopamine: insights from Parkinson's disease. Neuron 2009 ; 61 : 502-510.

74. Grant JE, Kim SW, Hollander E, Potenza MN. Predicting response to opiate antagonists and placebo in the treatment of pathological gambling. Psychopharmacology 2008;200 : 521-527.

75. Moore RY, Bloom FE (1979) Central catecholamine neuron systems: anatomy and physiology of the norepinephrine and epinephrine systems. Annu Rev Neurosci 2:113- 168.

76. Sofuoglu M, Sewell RA (2009) Norepinephrine and stimulant addiction. Addict Biol 14(2):119-129.

77. Drouin C, Darracq L, Trovero F, Blanc G, Glowinski J, Cotecchia S, Tassin JP (2002) Alpha1b-adrenergic receptors control locomotor and rewarding effects of psychostimulants and opiates. J Neurosci 22(7):2873-2884.

78. Themes UFO. 22: Pathological gambling and neurobiology I Medicine Key [Internet]. [cited 27 Apr 2024]. Available from: https://clemedicine.com/22-jeu-pathologique-et- neurobiology/

79. Pallanti S, Bernardi S, Allen A, Chaplin W, Watner D, DeCaria CM, Hollander E (2010) Noradrenergic function in pathological gambling: blunted growth hormone response to clonidine. J Psychopharmacol 24(6):847-853.

80. Bullock SA, Potenza MN (2012) Pathological gambling: neuropsychopharmacology and treatment. Curr Psychopharmacol 1(1):67-85.

81. Nordin C, Eklundh T (1999) Altered CSF 5-HIAA disposition in pathologic

male gamblers. CNS Spectr 4(12):25-33.

82. Marazziti D, Golia F, Picchetti M, Pioli E, Mannari P, Lenzi F, Conversano C, Carmassi C, Catena Dell'Osso M, Consoli G, Baroni S, Giannaccini G, Zanda G, Dell'Osso L (2008)
Decreased density of the platelet serotonin transporter in pathological gamblers. Neuropsychobiology 57(1-2):38-43.

83. Herz A (1997) Endogenous opioid systems and alcohol addiction. Psychopharmacology (Berl) 129(2):99-111.

84. Pecina S, Smith KS, Berridge KC (2006) Hedonic hot spots in the brain. Neuroscientist 12(6):500-511.
85. Spanagel R, Herz A, Shippenberg TS (1992) Opposing tonically active endogenous opioid systems modulate the mesolimbic dopaminergic pathway. Proc Natl Acad Sci U S A89(6):2046-2050.
86. Chen M, Sun Y, Lu L, Shi J. Similarities and Differences in Neurobiology. Adv Exp Med Biol. 2017;1010:45-58.

87. Grant J.E, Kim S.W, Odlaug B.L. N-acetyl cysteine, a glutamate-modulating agent, in the treatment of pathological gambling: a pilot study. Biol. Psychiatry. 2007;62:652-657.

88. Grant, J. E., Kim, S. W., Hollander, E. & Potenza, M. N. 2008 Predicting response to opiate antagonists and placebo in the treatment of pathological gambling. Psychopharmacology.

89. Chambers R.A, Bickel W.K, Potenza M.N. A scale-free systems theory of motivation and addiction. Neurosci. Biobehav. Rev. 2007;31:1017-1045.

90. Kalivas P.W, Volkow N.D. The neural basis of addiction: a pathology of motivation and choice. Am. J. Psychiatry. 2005;162:1403-1413.

91. Coric V, Kelmendi B, Pittenger C, Wasylink S, Bloch M.H. Beneficial

effects of the antiglutamatergic agent riluzole in a patient diagnosed with trichotillomania. J. Clin. Psychiatry. 2007;68:170-171.

92. Yau YHC, Potenza MN. Gambling Disorder and Other Behavioral Addictions: Recognition and Treatment. Harv Rev Psychiatry. 2015;23(2):134-46.

93. Kim SW, Grant JE, Adson DE, Shin YC. A double-blind comparative study of naltrexone and placebo in the treatment of pathological gambling. Biological Psychiatry. 2001 ; 49 : 914-921.

94. Grant JE, Potenza MN, Hollander E et al. Multicentre investigation of the antagonist opioid nalmefene in the treatment of pathological gambling. Suis J Psychiatry. 2006 ; 163 : 303-12.

95. A double-blind placebo-controlled study of the efficacy and safety of paroxetine in the treatment of pathological gambling. J Clin Psychiatry. 2002 ; 63 : 501-7.

96. Hollander E, DeCaria CM, Finkell JN, Begaz T, Wong CM, Cartwright C. A randomized double-blind fluvoxamine/placebo crossover trial in pathological gambling. Biol Psychiatry. 2000 ; 47 : 813-7.

97. Blanco C, Petkova E, Ibanez A, Saiz-Ruiz J. A placebo-controlled pilot study fluvoxamine for pathological gambling. Ann Clin Psychiatry. 2002 ; 14 : 9-15.

98. Grant JE, Potenza MN. Pharmacological Treatment of Adolescent Pathological Gambling. Int J Adolesc Med Health. 2010;22(1):129-38.

99. Grant JE, Kim SW, Potenza MN. Advances in the pharmacotherapy of pathological gambling. Journal of Gambling Studies. 2003;19:85-109.

100. Bullock SA, Potenza MN. Pathological Gambling: Neuropsychopharmacology and Treatment. Curr Psychopharmacol. Feb 1, 2012;1(1):10.2174/2211556011201010067.

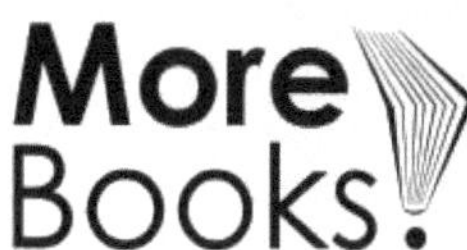

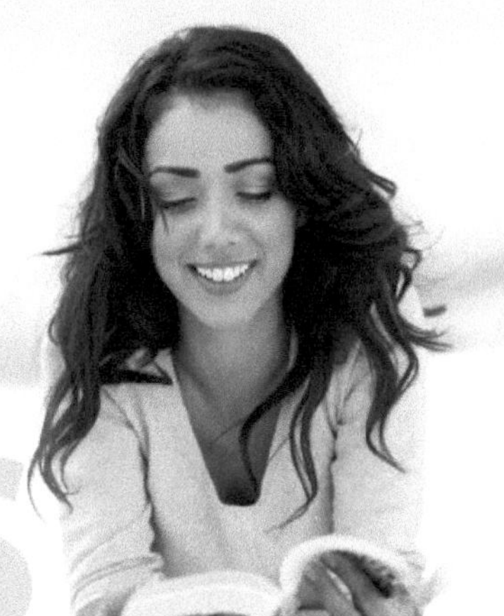

yes

I want morebooks!

Buy your books fast and straightforward online - at one of world's fastest growing online book stores! Environmentally sound due to Print-on-Demand technologies.

Buy your books online at

www.morebooks.shop

Kaufen Sie Ihre Bücher schnell und unkompliziert online – auf einer der am schnellsten wachsenden Buchhandelsplattformen weltweit! Dank Print-On-Demand umwelt- und ressourcenschonend produzi ert.

Bücher schneller online kaufen

www.morebooks.shop

info@omniscriptum.com
www.omniscriptum.com

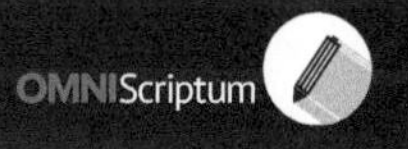

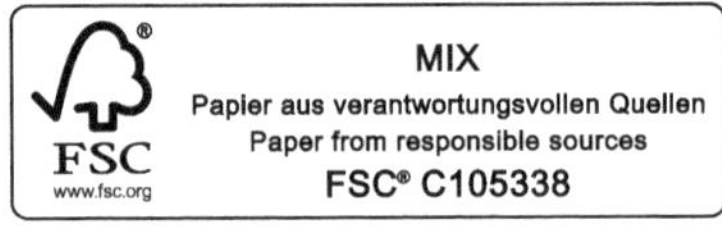

Printed by Books on Demand GmbH, Norderstedt / Germany